Recently Diagnosed With Diabetes: Tips for Managing

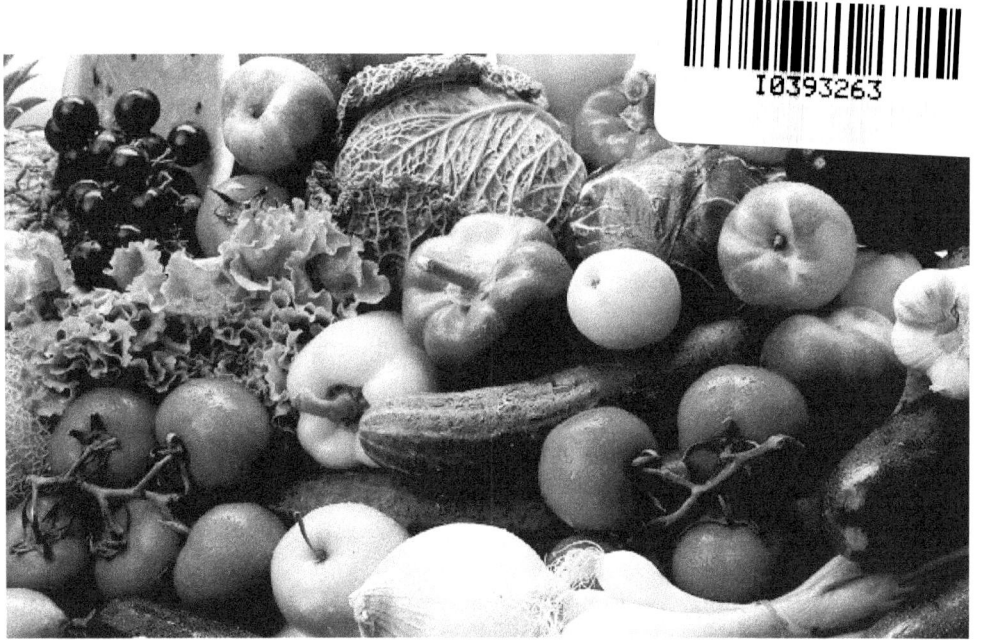

DISCLAIMER: This information is not presented by a medical practitioner and is for educational and informational purposes only. The content is not intended to be a substitute for professional medical advice, diagnosis, or treatment. Always seek the advice of your physician or other qualified health provider with any questions you may have regarding a medical condition.

Recently Diagnosed With Diabetes: Tips For Managing

A Global Epidemic

The Best Course of Action is Prevention

Prevention through Better Nutrition

Why Is It Called The Stealth Disease?

What Are the Symptoms?

Diabetes Defined - Type I and Type II Diabetes

Your Cardiovascular System and Diabetes

All about the Pancreas

Newly Diagnosed? Why you need a Nutritionist

Vitamins, Minerals and Supplements

Mealtime - Eat Protein Serving First

Mealtime - Eat Carbohydrate Serving Second

Mealtime - Eat Veggies and Grains Third

Obesity and Diabetes

Diet and Exercise

Diabetes - A Global Epidemic

When you hear the word epidemic, you may likely think of diseases that plague thousands of people in less developed countries far away. However, epidemics are not exclusive to such places. In fact, the world's most widespread epidemics strike a lot closer to home than what you may think.

An epidemic defined is a disease that has come to affect a large portion of a given population. The exact parameters differ among experts but a good estimation puts the number at around 3% of a population. Around 371 million people worldwide have Diabetes and 187 million of them do not even know they have the disease, according to the International Diabetes Federation (IDF).

Diabetes is now considered an epidemic that is affecting not just a select number of countries but the entire globe. It joins a short, but unfortunately, growing list of diseases of which, HIV/AIDS is part of. Projections for the disease's spread are alarming. The Center for Disease Control and Prevention has projected that as many as 1 in 3 U.S. adults will have diabetes by 2050 if current trends continue. An estimated 285 million people worldwide had diabetes in 2010, according to the International Diabetes Federation. The federation expects as many as 438 million will have diabetes by 2030.

The disease comes in two forms: Type I and Type II. Both, however, are similar in that both types involve the hormone insulin in the body and its ability to process sugar in the bloodstream. Too much or too little sugar in the body has adverse effects ranging from kidney failure, eyesight loss, and in extreme cases, coma.

Type I diabetes occurs when the immune system attacks the insulin forming cells in the body, misled into thinking that these cells are harmful. The pancreas therefore fail to produce insulin leading to a heightened level of sugar in the body, which puts stresses the kidneys, leading to further complications.

Most of the patients demonstrate the disease's symptoms at around 15 years of age, although the disease may have already been contracted years before. It is because of this that experts have interchanged the term Type I diabetes with "juvenile onset diabetes".
However, recently, this practice has been set aside in light of the alarmingly increasing number of young people contracting Type II

diabetes.

Type II diabetes (also known as "adult onset diabetes") is characterized by the body's failure to process sugar in the bloodstream despite the fact that insulin is produced by the pancreas. This could be because not enough insulin is produced or that the body simply does not respond to it. This form of diabetes accounts for 90 percent of the estimated 300 million cases of the disease worldwide.

There is a huge correlation between Type II diabetes and obesity. Most obese individuals lead a sedentary lifestyle, while consuming food high in carbohydrates, sugars and fat. These poor eating habits coupled with the lack / absence of physical activity increases the volume of sugar in the bloodstream. The pancreas cannot produce enough insulin to meet the demands of processing so much sugar and therefore diabetes sets in.

If left unchecked, the complications arising from diabetes are many and adverse.

- Retinopathy is the degeneration of the retina of the eye, leading to loss of sight.

- Kidney diseases / failure sets in when the organ finally breaks down due to the excessive stress from filtering too much sugar in the blood.

- Nervous system disorders are experienced by around half of diabetes sufferers. Symptoms such as impaired sensation in the limbs, carpal tunnel syndrome, and even impotence have been recorded among diabetics. When sensation is impaired in the limbs, infection from injuries may progress without being noticed, leading to no other resort but amputation.

- Diabetic coma (diabetic ketoacidosis) occurs when a patient becomes severely dehydrated and metabolism is greatly imbalanced. Since the cells in the body are starved of energy, the entire body shuts down leading to a coma.

These complications, however, pale in comparison to the number of lives that are lost every year due to diabetes. As of now, the number of deaths related to the disease is placed at around 4 million annually. But perhaps the greater tragedy is the fact that the adverse effect of diabetes (particularly with Type II) could have been prevented. But seen from a different point of view, that is also part of the good news. By observing a healthy lifestyle of eating and exercising right, the chances of leading a full and productive life despite the disease are very possible.

Start with the selection of the right food and its intake in the proper amounts. Consultation with a medical professional will inform you on what is right for your body type.

Observe the habit of physical exercises throughout the day. A regimented workout schedule may not be necessary. Walking and doing manual household chores may be sufficient. Again, consult with your doctor to know what is appropriate for you.

If you are diabetic, or at risk of it, or if you know someone who is, take the time to share this information and learn more about it. If the proper information and motivation is shared enough, there still may be a chance to reverse the tide of this global epidemic.

Taking a stand against Diabetes

Do you feel thirsty all the time? Do you frequently urinate? Do you have sores or wounds in your body that do not heal easily? Do you get tired easily? If you answered yes to most of these questions, then you might consider checking up with your doctor.

If you already have diabetes, then early detection can help you manage the disease. If you do not have diabetes, then it is time to eat and live right to prevent the disease from affecting you.

The previously mentioned conditions are some of the common symptoms of a chronic disease known as Diabetes. It is a serious illness which may not generally cause death, but can lead to more serious health problems that may lead to death.

Diabetes occurs when there is too much sugar or glucose in the bloodstream. Having this condition for a long period can lead to complications that may affect the body's important organs like the heart, eyes, and kidneys.

Diabetes can be classified as Type 1, Type 2 or Gestational.
Type 1 Diabetes affects both adults and children. Under this type, the body cannot properly use a hormone called insulin. The body's immune system harms the cells making insulin, resulting to low insulin level.

The condition of having a high sugar level with low insulin level can cause serious health problems.

Type 2 Diabetes can be managed with proper exercise and good eating habits. Maintaining an ideal weight is advisable because too much body fat and inactivity makes it harder for the body to use insulin. Under this type, the body is still able to make insulin but it cannot be used efficiently by the body.

Gestational Diabetes is found among pregnant women. This disease can make pregnancy more difficult than it already is. Those who are diagnosed with this type of Diabetes are at the high risk sector, of getting the second type. In normal pregnant women, their pancreas produces enough insulin that keeps the body's sugar level. However there are women whose pancreas are not able to produce enough insulin, resulting to gestational diabetes. Women with gestational diabetes need extra care, requiring a health diet and regular check ups. However, gestational diabetes usually disappears after giving birth and the baby is born without the disease. Among women who are at risk of gestational diabetes are those who are over 30 years old, have big babies during previous pregnancies, family history of diabetes and of course, the weight factor.

A person who has diabetes or is at risk of getting diabetes should start living a life that is geared towards diabetes prevention. To be able to do this, a person must know the factors that may be used to control or manage the disease.

Weight is an important factor in the control and management of diabetes, with those on the heavy side at a higher risk of getting diabetes. Keeping one's body fit and healthy is a sure way of avoiding diabetes and other diseases. This can be done by avoiding bad habits like smoking. One can also try to be m ore active by exercising regularly. Monitoring one's blood pressure is also important.

The good news is, one can avoid and prevent diabetes by resorting to a healthy lifestyle. However, there are factors that cannot be controlled and which can lead to getting diabetes, no matter what. One's heredity is an important factor in being a candidate for diabetes. And no matter how one keeps a healthy lifestyle, people who are 40 years old and above are at risk of getting Type 2 Diabetes. But then again, a healthy lifestyle will always help in preventing the disease.

A person who exhibits any of the symptoms of the disease or who belong to the high-risk group like having family members who have diabetes, should have himself examined by a doctor as soon as possible, Among the tests to assess a person's risks of getting diabetes are the glucose test, urine test, fasting plasma glucose test which measures the level of glucose in a person's blood after fasting for 12 to 14 hours, the oral glucose tolerance test which is also performed after fasting for three hours and the random plasma glucose test which can be done at any time.

The number of persons getting the disease has been increasing in the past years, due to poor eating habits, increasing inactivity and other factors that could have been prevented. Having yourself checked for diabetes can help you understand the disease. But no matter what you do to manage your diabetes, it would have been better if you were able to prevent it from affecting you.

Preventing Diabetes by Eating Right

An ounce of prevention is always better than cure, particularly if diabetes runs in your family. But this time, people need tons of prevention to keep this chronic disease from further seeping into the mainstream not only of the American society but also of societies all over the world.

Diabetes has become so widespread that the United States spends as much as $100 billion a year for the healthcare of Americans with diabetes. Millions of people all over the world have diabetes. The sad thing is most of them do not know they have it until it is too late.

Diabetes is a devastating disease which can damage the vital organs of the body including the kidneys, heart and the eyes. While diabetes does not really kill people, it can result to more serious and complicated diseases. Diabetes may not kill people as a general rule, but it makes them lose their eyesight, and leads them to kidney and heart problems, and later on, death.

People with diabetes can survive the diseases provided they practice proper health care. Those who do not have the disease, but are in danger of getting the disease due to heredity, can avoid getting the Big D through proper nutrition.

Aside from heredity, the top cause of diabetes is improper diet. Modern man's propensity for leading hectic lives has led them into eating the wrong kinds of food. Man has become so obsessed with wealth creation and pleasure, that he has no more time to prepare a well-balanced meal. Thus, the modern man's diet consists of canned goods, processed fish, meat and vegetables that can be eaten immediately by just popping it inside a microwave. The modern world has convinced man to have a preference for refined food, from sugar to grains.

Most people who are healthy all their lives are getting diabetes and the culprit is the kind of food they eat, and our ignorance as to the nutrient content of the food we eat.

But there are health-friendly foods that are available in the market, one only has to learn how to recognize and eat them. It's just a matter of changing our choice of food, like preferring whole grains over refined grains such as brown rice, whole wheat bread and the likes. Eat more fruits and vegetables and less meat, sweet and oily food. It also helps to read the labels of processed food, to determine the amount of one's carbohydrate intakes.

Most people shy away from eating right because of the misconception about proper dieting. It is okay to eat certain kinds of food but you need to know how to eat them properly like knowing the proper number of servings, or the better way of cooking such food. If you find vegetables boring, then be creative in your food preparation. Differently colored salads can encourage your good appetite.

If you can't resist oily food, then avoid going to fast food joints because seeing french-fries hungry people will just make your saliva drop and will make you forget you diet.

So how does one know that he already has diabetes? The common symptoms are frequent urination, fatigue and being thirsty all the time. Diabetes simply means too much glucose in your bloodstream. Too much glucose in the body requires more water, thus making you feel thirsty most of the time. With thirst comes an increased water intake, making urination frequent.

The other symptoms of diabetes includes an increase or decrease in weight, blurred vision, sores or wounds that are slow to heal and sometimes lead to infections and tender gums.

Obesity makes one at a greater risk of getting diabetes so it is also important to watch your weight. Those who have excess fat in the belly are more prone to being health risks. Weight gain or about 10 to 20 pounds, no matter how moderate, can also make one a candidate for diabetes.

Aside from eating the right food and watching one's weight, it is also good to increase one's physical activity. It does not necessarily mean you have to become a sportsman all of a sudden. Gardening, although a mild physical activity, can help you relax and lose weight as well. Try ball catching or ball kicks with your children, it is not only a good way to bond but is also a way to lose those extra fats.

Eating is such a pleasure, particularly if you know how to eat right.

Why Is It Called The Stealth Disease?

Stealth, by definition, is the way of moving without being seen, felt or detected. Does diabetes exhibit these characteristics to be tagged as the stealth disease?

Diabetes is a chronic disease in which the level of blood glucose of a person is higher than normal. There are several symptoms that tell a person he has diabetes. Some of these are frequent urination accompanied by unusual thirst, dramatic change in weight, blurring of vision, lack of energy, and many more. However, not all people who actually have diabetes show these symptoms. Diabetes can already be quietly creeping inside your system without you
knowing it, especially on its early stages. According to the
statistics, currently one in ten US adults of have diabetes right now.

Different Forms of Diabetes

There are three different types of diabetes – Type I, Type II, and Gestational diabetes. We discussed Type I and II previously as juvenile and adult. Let's review the first two types.
Formerly known as the juvenile diabetes, Type 1 is usually diagnosed at a younger age, mostly during childhood. This type can be linked to the person's genes. In this type, the pancreas has stopped producing insulin. Thus, in order for a Type 1 diabetic to survive, he needs to continuously take insulin shots.

Type 2 diabetes, also known as the adult-onset diabetes, is most common among diabetic patients – almost 90% of diabetic patients have this type. From the term adult-onset, this type of diabetes is mostly diagnosed at a later age in life. Some may have had it since childhood but just didn't realize until later. This is because, most of the time, type 2 diabetes starts to show symptoms when it is already in the advanced stage.

Type 2 diabetes can also be linked to the person's lifestyle and diet. That is why people who are overweight or those aged 40 and above have greater risks in developing this type of the disease. Thus, to control or prevent having diabetes in the future, we should all be mindful of the things we do and the food we eat.

The third kind is the gestational diabetes. This is only present in pregnant women, most of the time during the third trimester. This kind is usually caused by certain hormones brought about by pregnancy or, like the other types, lack of insulin. Ob-Gyns oftentimes require their patients to undergo the Oral Glucose Tolerance Test, especially when the woman is almost overweight due to her pregnancy. Even if this type ceases after giving birth, there is a big possibility that the woman will acquire Type 2 diabetes in the future.

If no proper care is administered or left improperly managed, this stealth disease can lead to further complications. These complications may be heart, kidney or eye problems, impotence or even nerve damage. Therefore, careful management is really necessary for diabetic patients.

How to Fight this Stealth Disease?

The first way to prevent diabetes, and probably the most important, is early diagnosis. The earlier this disease is diagnosed in your system, the sooner you can take action in managing it and, in turn, prevent further complications. The Canadian Diabetes Association actually recommends citizens over 40 years old to do regular screening every three years, and those with other high risk factors to do it every year.

Having a healthy lifestyle with regular exercise combined with a healthy diet is also one way of preventing, or managing, diabetes especially Type 2. Any disease, in fact, can be prevented if one focuses on staying and living healthy.

Diabetes, actually, is much better to manage now than years before. It is because people are now well educated about this condition. There have been several studies and researches done as well to continuously learn more about diabetes and find more ways in managing and controlling it.

Being conscious about the condition, proper management, continuous medication, and a healthy lifestyle are the keys to really prevent this condition from further aggravating and decrease the possibility of much more complications.

What Are the Symptoms of Diabetes?

Someone who is addicted to sugar or sweets is not necessarily a diabetic. Diabetes is a serious illness brought about by a person's genetic disposition: his likelihood to develop a pancreatic disease. If your family is prone to the disease, read this article to detect the symptoms of diabetes as early as possible.

Type I Diabetes
Type I is known as insulin-dependent diabetes mellitus (IDDM). It is less common in the US though is the most severe and usually develops within a few days or weeks. In IDDM, the lack of insulin stems from destruction of the beta cells. The symptoms associated with IDDM are so distinct that they rarely leave any doubt of the diagnosis.

They are as follows:

Polyuria: Urinating frequently and in large amounts is a classic symptom of diabetes, as the body rushes fluids through the kidney to dilute the high levels of sugar in the urine.

Polydipsia: An unusual thirst is a natural result of too frequent urination: the body is signaling for lost fluids to be replaced. Dehydration will eventually occur if the condition is not caught early.

Polyphagia: This feeling of extreme hunger stems from the body's belief that it is starving because glucose is not reaching its cells to provide desperately needed energy.
Rapid Weight Loss: Most Type I patients are at or below their ideal weight. When IDDM begins, they may suddenly lose more weight—as much as 15 pounds in a week—even though they may be eating more than enough and have a good appetite. The lack of insulin means that calories, in the form of glucose, are being sent out through the urine and the body is beginning to burn fat reserves.

Weakness: Since muscle cells are not receiving their usual fuel, energy flags. Of course, fatigue can have many causes, which is why diabetes can go unrecognized for so long. Be concerned if a once active child seems tired, drowsy, or listless for no apparent reason. Some children may also complain of stomach, leg, or chest pains, or have difficulty breathing.

Irritability: In youngsters, crankiness, confusion or excessive crying may warn of impending illness. A child may seem to be inattentive or may not be doing as well in school as before.

Nausea and/or Vomiting: These symptoms may precede ketoacidosis, as poisonous ketone acids build up in the blood when the body must resort to burning fat deposits for energy.

Blurred Vision: Excess glucose may be seeping into the eye, changing the shape of the lens. Difficulty in focusing or changes in eyesight from one day to the next—such as from nearsighted to normal vision—are other visual cues for possible diabetes.

TYPE II
Type II, or non-insulin-dependent diabetes mellitus (NIDDM), makes up the majority of diabetes cases, estimated that about 13 million people in the US. Unlike Type I, Type II progresses more slowly. It can creep along unnoticed for years. Symptoms may appear gradually, becoming more intense or frequent with age.

See your doctor as soon as you observe any of the following:

Any of Type I symptoms

Tingling or Numbness in Legs, Feet, or Fingers: Or you may have a burning sensation or heightened sensitivity in these extremities or on other spots on your skin. Symptoms, such as leg cramps, may appear or worsen only at night. Again, these may be signs that circulation is poor or that nerve damage is already progressing.

Frequent Infections: Diabetes weakens the body's defenses against invasions of bacteria. Infections of the gums, urinary tract, or skin that keep recurring or take a long time to clear up show that the disease may have begun interfering with the immune system.

Itching of Skin or Genitals: This may be the result of an underlying infection or dehydration, a common by-product of diabetes.

Slow Healing of Cuts and Bruises: Because diabetes affects how cells use the nutrients obtained from food, the body may have difficulty repairing damaged tissue. Diabetes also thickens blood vessels, slowing circulation and preventing wounds from receiving, through the blood, these needed nutrients and oxygen.

Unfortunately, too many of these symptoms can be overlooked or blamed on other conditions. Make sure to have your blood sugar level checked yearly, at the very least, and more frequently if there are manifestations of any of the symptoms above.

Diabetes Defined - Type I and Type II Diabetes

The word diabetes is a familiar one with most people. Unfortunately, its familiarity stems from the fact that so many people have been afflicted with this disease.

The disease is characterized by the body's impaired ability or failure to process glucose (a form of sugar) in the bloodstream because of the lack / absence of insulin. Insulin is a hormone produced in the pancreas that processes blood sugar into a form that the cells in the body can use for energy.

Without the proper processing of sugar, the body either becomes hyperglycemic (too much sugar) or hypoglycemic (too little sugar). Both are dangerous as it can make the body react in any number of ways such as weakened kidneys, impaired nervous system, loss of sight and in some extreme cases, coma.

Diabetes takes on two kinds of forms, and they differ from each other primarily through the means by which the disease is contracted.
The first type of diabetes (Type I) is contracted genetically. Most of the patients of this type are boys and girls of around 15 years old. It is because of this trend that experts have interchanged the term Type I diabetes with Juvenile Onset Diabetes.

The disease works by fooling the body's immune system into thinking that the cells responsible for producing insulin are harmful. The islets of Langerhans (as these cells are called) are attacked by the immune system, rendering the islets unable to produce the necessary hormone to process blood sugar.

Diabetics of this type need to have insulin administered regularly into their system. As of now, the most common method for delivering the hormone is through injections. Other delivery systems are also being developed, the most recent of which is an oral spray that eliminates the need for hypodermic needles. This measure simply manages the condition but does not fully address the problem of curing it.

Short of a pancreas transplant, there is no cure for Type I diabetes. And even then, the risks are considerable making anyone think twice before undergoing the procedure. This is because transplanted organs run the risk of being rejected by the recipient's body even if blood types match. However, should the transplant prove successful, the diabetic may no longer have the need to have insulin artificially introduced into his / her body. A trade off exists in that in order to prevent organ rejection, the patient will have to take immuno-suppressive drugs throughout their lifetime, which may make him / her more susceptible to infections than usual.

Even then, most patients who have undergone the procedure say that it is a price they are willing to pay in exchange for a life free of needles and in fear of the complications the disease brings.

Type II diabetes
Of the total number of cases of diabetes worldwide, Type II accounts for more than 90 percent. Until recently, Type II diabetes was also called Adult Onset Diabetes, with the average age of a symptomatic patient around 40 years of age. But the increasing number of cases of children acquiring this type of the disease has led experts into setting this term aside.

Type II diabetes is characterized by the body's impaired ability / failure to process sugar despite the presence of insulin-producing cells. The pancreas cannot keep up with the demand to produce enough insulin to process sugar in the body.
The cause for Type II diabetes is a lot less ominous than the first one. Whereas Type I is genetic, where the patient has no control over it, the second type of diabetes is usually brought about by a lifestyle of poor eating and exercise habits.

Doctors and research scientists alike are finding more and more the direct proportion of obesity to Type II diabetes. Findings show that overweight and obese individuals are very likely to contract the disease and their chances of succumbing to the complications brought by the disease increase significantly.

This is perhaps what makes Type II diabetes such an alarming situation. Many experts feel that the number of people living
with this disease need not be as great had they observed proper diet and exercise.

To manage the disease, Type II diabetics are instructed to exercise regularly, limit their carbohydrate and sugar intake and when absolutely necessary, have insulin administered artificially.

More research is done to resolve the disease and each step brings medicine closer to a solution. But for now the good news lies in that with proper care and observance of the instructions, a diabetic of either the first or second type can still live a full and productive life.

Your Cardiovascular System and Diabetes

Cardiovascular system is one of the most important systems in the human body. It is comprised of the heart, blood and blood vessels. Blood is being pumped out from the heart and is the one responsible in delivering oxygen and other nutrients to all the parts of the body. It also cleans up our body by picking up the waste products on its way back to the heart so our body can get rid of them.

So what has diabetes got to do with the cardiovascular system? Since blood is part of the cardiovascular system, and diabetes is a condition in which the level of glucose in the blood is higher than normal, then there must be some relationship between the two.

Diabetes and cardiovascular system diseases has been recognized to be closely related to each other for some time now due to the so-called insulin resistance syndrome or metabolic syndrome.
Some examples of the commonly diagnosed cardiovascular disease are coronary heart disease, stroke, high blood pressure and other heart conditions.

Cardiovascular diseases are the major cause now of deaths related to diabetes. In a study published few years back in the Journal of the American Medical Association, deaths due to some heart conditions went up by 23% in diabetic women despite the 27% drop of the same in nondiabetic women.

As for diabetic men, there is only about 13% decrease in heart disease related deaths as compared to the 36% drop in nondiabetics.

Thus, the two indeed go together.

Risk Factors

Diabetes is now considered by the American Heart Association a major risk factor in cardiovascular diseases. Other factors that contribute to the possibility of acquiring cardiovascular diseases in diabetic patients include hypertension, smoking, and dyslipidemia.

- Hypertension. Hypertension in diabetes is considered a major contributor to the increase in mortality from cardiovascular diseases.

Diabetic patients, especially those with Type 2, need to always have their blood pressure checked every visit to the doctor. Self-monitoring at home is also a must to maintain and control the rise of blood pressure. The American Diabetes Association recommends a target blood pressure of not more than 130/85 mm Hg to maintain a good level of blood pressure.

- Hyperglycemia. Intensive glycemic control may prove to reduce the risk of cardiovascular events, although not directly. This can be more beneficial in controlling micro vascular complications, but still, assessing all risk factors and properly managing them is a big step in preventing occurrence of any cardiovascular diseases.

- Smoking. Smoking has been determined dangerous to our health. Studies show that smoking indeed increase risk of premature death and cardiovascular disease in diabetic patients.

Prevention
As the old saying goes, "prevention is better than cure." There are many ways on how to prevent the increased possibility of cardiovascular events in diabetic patients. Several alterations or modifications to the risk factors can be done to still maintain healthy despite of diabetes.

The simplest step one can start with is to stop smoking. Diabetic or not, cessation of smoking will really prove beneficial to one's overall health condition. Maintaining blood pressure to less than 130/85 or 130/80 mm Hg helps control the occurrence of hypertension. Having a body mass index (BMI) of less than 27 is also a must for diabetic patients to control their overall condition.

Some tests are also recommended to monitor and keep maintain key factors at a healthy level. These tests include annual urine test, retinal dilation examination, dental examinations, and biannual foot examination for sensation testing and measurement of pulses. Influenza and pnuemococcal immunizations also help in proper maintenance.

Diabetes and cardiovascular diseases need proper attention and care. Regular visits to your health practitioner are recommended as they are the right people who know all about your condition. They keep all the records of their patients' health history and can track improvements or otherwise. Proper medications and advice are also given by these professionals.

Diabetes is indeed a life-long condition that demands a lot of attention. There may be no hard and real cure for this disease, but it sure can be maintained and controlled by proper care and having thorough knowledge and understanding about the condition.

All about the Pancreas and Diabetes

Diabetes ranks among the top 10 causes of death in most developed and industrialized societies. But what is diabetes and how does it affect the body?

Diabetes is a disease that stems from the lack of insulin. Insulin is a hormone produced by the body to process glucose. Glucose is a form of sugar that the cells of the body need for energy. But before a cell can use glucose, insulin is needed to process the sugar into a form the cell can absorb.

Without insulin, the cells do not the energy needed to run the body properly, making a person weak. Furthermore, since the glucose is not used up it stays in the blood, which is harmful to the body, particularly to the kidneys.

Without proper treatment, the complications arising from diabetes are many and severe. Some of these include eyesight loss (retinopathy), nerve damage, kidney failure, and in very severe cases, diabetic ketoacidosis (diabetic coma).

There are two types of diabetes, differing in cause of contracting the disease, but nevertheless both are equally serious. Type I diabetes is caused by the body's immune system mistakenly attacking the cells responsible for the production of insulin. As these cells are destroyed, insulin production is halted as well.

Type II diabetes is primarily caused by the body's inability to process glucose even if insulin is present in the body. This is mainly because there is too much sugar in the body and not enough insulin is produced to process the excess sugar. As such, the blood sugar levels rise while putting extreme stress on the pancreas.

The pancreas is a gland that lies crosswise and behind the stomach. It is where insulin is produced and released into the body. Cells called islets of Langerhans are the primary makers of insulin, and these are what the immune system attacks in a Type I diabetes case.

In the case of Type II diabetes, the pancreas is forced to produce so much insulin to cope with the high levels of sugar in the body.

Unfortunately, if high sugar levels are maintained for long periods of time, the undue stress may cause the pancreas to break down.

Most Type I diabetic patients manage the disease by having insulin artificially administered. The most common methods are pills and hypodermic needle syringes. Other delivery methods are being developed as well, such as an oral spray that delivers the patient's required amount of insulin.

Those with Type II diabetes may not need artificial insulin administration. A different medication can be coupled with a controlled diet and exercise. As there is a proven correlation between Type II diabetes and obesity, doctors and health experts recommend obese individuals to undergo a regimented weight loss and management program to combat the disease. However, in advanced cases of Type II diabetes, artificial insulin administration could be prescribed.

For Type I diabetes, no real cure exists, except for a pancreatic transplant. Since the patient's own pancreas has been compromised by the diseases, new pancreas is needed to restore the body's own ability to produce insulin.

There already have been reported and successful cases of pancreatic transplants, but the risks and stakes are very high. The chances are great that the body's immune system may reject the new part leading to very serious and fatal complications.

Furthermore, research shows that a good number of those successful pancreatic transplants involved having undergone a kidney transplant as well. The mortality rate of patients who've undergone just the transplant of the pancreas is greater compared to cases of patients who'd undergone pancreas and kidney transplants.

Prevention of diabetes is highly possible, and extremely easy if you already are observing proper dietary and exercise habits.

If, however, you find yourself leading a lifestyle with little physical activity while consuming food high in sugar, you should take stock of your current lifestyle and seriously consider changing. Consult with a doctor to help you assess your current state as far as diabetes is concerned. The sooner these are done, the better. As you become kinder to your body, it will respond accordingly.

Newly Diagnosed? Why you need a Nutritionist

One of the most important things that people who have just been diagnosed with diabetes have to pay attention to is their dietary plan. They have to make sure that they have a proper diet. This will help them maintain good health, and well being!

It is a must for people who have diabetes to acquire the assistance of a nutritionist. This is because every individual that has diabetes requires a dietary plan that is customized to suit their needs. A good nutritionist will be able to assess the type of meal that an individual needs depending on what type of health concerns he/she might have.

Those people who need to shed some pounds will benefit greatly from nutritionists. A nutritionist will be able to help them come up with a dietary plan that will help them lose weight, while maintaining the nutrients that their body needs.

Carbohydrates

Most carbohydrates that are introduced into the body are turned into glucose. What happens is that the glucose goes into the body's blood stream. This in turn causes the body to release insulin. What insulin does is it causes glucose to go from the bloodstream into the cells, where it will then become a stored energy source.

The important thing is to achieve a proper balance between the carbohydrates, having enough exercise and the right amount of insulin. This is to make sure that the blood sugar level in the body remains regulated.

Regulate your meals

To help maintain healthy sugar level individuals should regulate their meals. This means as much as possible, try to eat meals at the same time each day.

After eating, a person's blood glucose escalates. If a person eats a huge meal one day and eats a light meal the next, his or her blood sugar level will become unstable.

Carbohydrates when absorbed turns into glucose. Individuals must keep track of the amount of carbohydrates that they consume. They can do this by reading food labels. Carbohydrates are usually measured in grams.

Also, it would be best if individuals try to consume the same amount of food for every meal. Another thing that is important is not to skip meals.

For the best possible method of regulating one's diet, those who have diabetes should consult their doctors. They will be able to provide a proper meal plan that would be specifically designed to meet the needs of each and every individual.
Support System

Those who are newly diagnosed with diabetes can enter hospital programs where they are educated about the disease. They are also informed about new dietary plans, and changes they need to incorporate into their lifestyle to lead a healthy life.

People who have just discovered that they have diabetes need a strong support system. During this time they might feel extremely vulnerable. They would need emotional support. This is the time where family and friends come in handy. Especially during the time they are still adjusting and discovering ways to come to terms with their new health condition.

Vitamins, Minerals and Supplements against Diabetes

Diabetes is a serious illness affecting America over the last decade. Though it is a well-known disease, there is no cure for it; but only management, to prevent worsening the condition and further complications. There are two categories of diabetes.

Type I is known as insulin-dependent diabetes mellitus (IDDM). In IDDM, the lack of insulin stems from destruction of the beta cells that prevent the body from producing insulin. It usually occurs early in life, during childhood, and the young patient is made to live with a lifetime of insulin injections.

Type II, or non-insulin-dependent diabetes mellitus (NIDDM), makes up the majority of diabetes cases, estimated that about 13 million people in the US. Unlike Type I, the pancreas of Type II patients eventually wears out, and no longer produces sufficient insulin that is recognized by the body. It can creep along unnoticed for years, and is usually diagnosed when one is an adult (25 years old above).

Based on the two types, it seems that only the administration of insulin is the only solution to the management of the disease. However, recent studies show that insulin is not alone in combating the diabetes. Here are a few significant vitamins, minerals and supplements against diabetes.

Vitamin D

Vitamin D is a nutrient found in the body that contains calcium and phosphorus, chemicals needed for bone growth and strength. It is formed on the skin, when cholesterol at the subcutaneous level interacts with the ultraviolet rays of the sun. Traditionally known as the nutrient to combat osteoporosis (bones becoming brittle due to loss of calcium), Vitamin D has been tested and found to prevent diabetes as well.

A research conducted in Finland, where people are exposed to very little sunlight, proved that Vitamin D protected children against high blood sugar, a first sign of diabetes. The experiment was conducted on 12,000 children who were administered Vitamin D from birth (1966).

Researchers published in 2012 that they have observed that 80% of the risks for diabetes were reduced, mainly preventing high blood sugar, than that of those that did not receive Vitamin D supplements.

However, Endocrinologists desire more validation for this result because they have found no correlation yet between the efficacies of the Vitamin with the nature of diabetes. They also caution that too much of Vitamin D is toxic, thus the administration must be under the supervision of a doctor.

Vitamin E

Next up in the alphabet, Vitamin E. For the past decade, health and nutrition experts have concluded that antioxidants help combat free radicals, bad cells in the body that cause diseases like cancer and type II diabetes, together with a healthy diet and lifestyle. Well, since type II diabetes is a condition of voluntary cell dysfunction, antioxidants can help in this aspect. Antioxidants include among others, Vitamin E.

Vitamin E is a fat-soluble nutrient found in milk, plant leaves and wheat germ oil. It has been proven to aid reproduction in both lab experiments and actual human experience. A widely used form of Vitamin E, alpha-tocopherol is ingested into the body in the form of gel capsules. Though its effect in diabetes prevention is real, an increase in the vitamin intake was not proven to be proportional to the level of prevention.

Minerals

Minerals are inorganic nutrients that are essential in normal bodily functions as well as combat diseases, like diabetes.

Magnesium and potassium are minerals that aid in carbohydrate and protein metabolism. The proper breakdown and synthesis of carbohydrate into simple sugars is a function that diabetics lack. With the aid of the two minerals, it can help prevent the disease. Chromium and zinc facilitate the recognition of insulin in the body.

Supplements

A third type of nutrient that fight diabetes is organic supplements. Blueberry is a fruit that is rich in antioxidants, which can address free radicals that cause body cells to malfunction. They particularly improve sight, which can help alleviate diabetic blindness.

Mamordica Charantia (bitter melon) is a vegetable that is rich in nutrients that enhance the production of beta cells, thus improving insulin production by the pancreas. In the Philippines, where the plant originates, it is a recommended supplement. Chinese herbal medicine also swears by this plant and actually uses it traditionally to address sterility, skin diseases and gastro-intestinal diseases. If one is able to tolerate the bitter taste, then it promises a high chance of improving pancreatic activity (by as much as 54%).

Coupled with a sensible diet and healthy lifestyle, using vitamins, minerals and supplements like the ones above, can help fight diabetes.

Eat protein serving first to prevent diabetes

Do you know that the number of individuals acquiring diabetes, particular Type 2 diabetes or adult onset diabetes is increasing? Makes this news more alarming is the fact that diabetes nowadays is not only hitting adults. There are even some reports suggesting that young people and children are acquiring diabetes. Around sixteen million individuals in the country are suffering from diabetes according to the United States Centers for Disease Control and Prevention.

Much has been said about the link between a high carb diet and diabetes but very little is documented about the connection between protein and diabetes. In fact, the role of protein in the diet of people at risk or suffering from diabetes has been marred in controversy. According old studies, most of the protein consumed was converted to glucose in the liver and raises blood glucose level as it entered the bloodstream.

Like carbohydrate, protein is also converted into glucose by a process called gluconeogenesis. And also similarly, the speed of this process depends on the amount of insulin secreted by the pancreas and the blood glucose control.

According to the same old studies, diabetic individuals convert protein to glucose very rapidly which can lead to a very negative effect on blood glucose level. In healthy, normal individuals, the intake of protein can stimulate insulin release as much as carbohydrates can. This has led experts to believe that eating protein does not help avoid hypoglycemia.

However, new studies have shown that while and estimated 50% to 60% of protein consumed is converted to glucose, it does not enter the bloodstream and thus does not raise the rate of glucose discharge by the liver. Nobody has yet to discover where the glucose goes. One theory speculates that it is probably stored in the liver or muscles as glycogen. But experts agree that it is least likely to affect blood glucose levels.

Now it is recommended hat people at with or at risk of acquiring diabetes includes more protein in their diets. The suggested amount of protein is 15 to 20 percent of the daily calorie intake. The protein however should be distributed throughout all the meals. In eating animal protein, one should make sure to choose only the lean parts and combine them with non-animal protein like those found in vegetables.

The amount of protein intake must not increase 20 percent of calories though as this may lead to the development of kidney disease. People with kidney problems should reduce the amount of protein intake to slow down or halt the progression of the disease.

One way to include more protein in your diet to prevent diabetes is to have protein servings first during mealtime then have carbohydrate rich foods served second.

An advantage of having protein serving first during mealtime is that it can reduce the amount of carbohydrate intake of your body. The logic here is that you would already fill full after the serving of protein so you would have less inclination to consume carbohydrates.

Individuals who have diabetes or who are at risk of getting the disease do not have the ability to process carbohydrates particularly sugars

properly. This is why a diet high in carbohydrates has always been linked to an increased risk of diabetes. Individuals suffering from diabetes and those who believe they are at a moderate or high risk of getting the disease must carefully follow a diet regimen that is low in carbohydrates. This is to ensure that their sugar levels would not be affected by an increase intake of carbs.
One simple fact that people should remember about carbohydrates is that they all break down into simple sugars. Whether you are eating complex carbohydrates like brown rice or whole wheat bread or you are consuming simple sugars like candies and white sugar, they would all end up as simple sugars inside your body.

Complex and simple carbohydrates differ only in the rate at which they are converted to basic sugars. Carbohydrates are converted to simple sugars from five minutes to 3 hours after consumption. Complex carbohydrate breaks down slower than simple sugars. This means that the impact of simple sugars and complex carbohydrates in the blood sugar level of individuals differs.

Individuals must therefore take note of their daily carbohydrate consumption in order to prevent diabetes. This is a very important thing to do if you really do not want to raise your blood sugar level. A good and effective way to achieve this is to eat protein serving first during mealtime.

To help prevent diabetes, eat carb serving second

The number of individuals acquiring diabetes, particular Type 2 diabetes or adult onset diabetes is increasing. This fact is very alarming. What is worse is that diabetes is not only hitting adults. There are even some reports suggesting that even young people and children are acquiring diabetes. The United States Centers for Disease Control and Prevention said that around sixteen million individuals in the country are suffering from diabetes.

A diet high in carbohydrates has always been linked to an increased risk of diabetes. This is because people who have diabetes or who are at risk of getting the disease do not have the ability to process carbohydrates particularly sugars properly. Individuals suffering from diabetes and those who believe they are at a moderate or high risk of getting the disease must carefully follow a diet plan that is low in carbohydrates. The level of carbohydrates can definitely have a large impact in ones blood sugar levels.

One way to reduce the amount of carbohydrates intake is to have carbohydrate servings second during mealtime. The first servings of food during mealtime should be composed of food low in carbohydrates or high in fiber or protein.

All carbohydrates break down into simple sugars. This is one fact that people should keep in mind. It doesn't matter if you are eating complex carbohydrates like brown rice or whole wheat bread or simple sugars like candies and white sugar, they would all end up the same inside your body.

So the important thing is to take note of your total carbohydrates intake. Counting carbohydrate and reduce its intake is therefore a must to prevent diabetes. And one effective way of doing this is to eat carb serving second during mealtime.

What is different between complex and simple carbohydrates is the rate at which they are converted into basic sugars. Carbohydrates are converted to simple sugars from five minutes to 3 hours after consumption. Complex carbohydrate breaks down slower than simple sugars. Therefore, the effect of complex carbohydrates and simple sugars in the blood sugar level of individuals varies quite differently.

It is also important to note that high fiber foods are usually low in sugars. This is why high intake of fiber can also greatly reduce the risk of diabetes. People who are at risk of getting diabetes are advised to increase their fiber intake by taking fiber supplements such as psyllium , guar gum, oat bran or glucomannan. They should also consume more vegetables, fruits, whole wheat products and whole grain products.

So what is the basis of a low carb diet? A low carb diet is based on the fact that fatty acids in the blood are stored in the body as fat in the fat cells because of the secretion of insulin. For those who still do not know, insulin is a hormone produce by the body and is secreted by the pancreas.

The difference between a healthy individual and someone suffering from diabetes is that the body of the former has the ability to properly take note of the amount of sugar circulated within it. Insulin is immediately secreted by the body of a normal healthy person when blood sugar suddenly increases. The role of insulin is to send a message to the fat cells in the body to absorb the triglycerides and glucose in the blood.

When glucose and triglycerides is absorbed by the fat cells, the blood sugar level returns to safe and normal levels. Diabetics have a problem with producing sufficient amounts of insulin. Some diabetics cannot produce any insulin at all.

You must also be familiar with the concept of glycemic Index. The ability of different foods to raise blood sugar varies and is measured through the glycemic index. Starchy, high carbohydrates foods raise the blood sugar and have a high glycemic index. The idea behind low carb diets is to keep blood sugar low so your body won't secrete significant quantities of insulin which in turn wouldn't put blood sugars and triglycerides into your fat cells.

And one of the ways to achieve this is to eat carb serving second during mealtime. This will ensure that by the time that the serving of carbohydrates come you will already be half full. Therefore you wouldn't eat as much as you would have if the carbohydrate serving was served first.

Eating More Vegetables and Whole Grains Will Help Prevent Diabetes

Medical findings have discovered that eating whole grain products might help prevent diabetes. This is due to the effect that after eating grounded grain, for example: flour, pastas, pastries, etc., the body experiences an escalation in blood sugar. While on the other hand, eating whole grain products does not make the body sugar rise as much.

Medical experts have found a healthy diet rich in whole grains will help prevent type 2 diabetes.

All about carbohydrates

Carbohydrates are categorized into two sections. Sugars and Starches. Most carbohydrates that is introduced into the body is turned into glucose. What happens is that the glucose goes into the body's blood stream. This in turn causes the body to release insulin. What insulin does is it causes glucose to go from the bloodstream into the cells, where it will then become stored energy source.

The important thing is to achieve a proper balance between the intake of carbohydrates, right amount of exercise and insulin level that goes into the system. This is to make sure that the blood sugar level in the body remains regulated.

Whole grains are good for you

Instead of using bleached or white flours, individuals who have diabetes should turn to whole grains instead. Whole grain products are by far healthier. They help maintain a good blood sugar level, since they do not make the level of blood sugar in the bloodstream rise so much.

Maintain a balanced diet

This means a lot of fruits and vegetables, and not burgers and fries! Fried foods are high in calories and fat! A healthy diet includes: food rich in fiber, whole grains, legumes, nuts, fruits and vegetables. Consumption of poultry products should be regulated. The use of salt should also be measured. Also they should drink plenty of water.

The way you eat affects how your body functions

To help maintain a healthy blood sugar level individuals should regulate their meals. This means as much as possible, try to eat meals at the same time each day. It would also be best if they try to consume the same amount of food for every meal After eating, a person's blood glucose escalates. If a person eats a huge meal one day and eats a light meal the next, his or her blood sugar level will become unstable. Also it would not be beneficial for those who have diabetes to skip meals. Carbohydrates when absorbed turns into glucose. Individuals must keep track of the amount of carbohydrates that they consume. They can do this by reading food labels. Carbohydrates are usually measured in grams.

It has been discovered that eating 5 to 6 small meals a day, is healthier than eating loads of food at one sitting.

For the best possible method of regulating one's diet. Individuals who have diabetes should consult a nutritionist. They will be able to provide a proper meal plan, that would be specifically designed to meet the needs of each and every individual!

Nutritionist

It is important to consult a nutritionist because every person that has diabetes requires a custom made dietary plan. One that is suited to promote good health. There are those individuals who have dietary needs that require special attention.

Those who need to lose some pounds will benefit greatly from the assistance of a nutritionist. A nutritionist would be able to come up with a plan that would help individuals lose weight, while maintaining a healthy and balanced diet.

Food Journal

It would not be a bad idea for people who have diabetes to list down all the foods that they eat per day. This is to keep track of all the food products they are consuming. So they would be aware of the types of nutrients that are going into their system. This will help them to maintain a healthy balance and balanced diet. Also, keeping a record would help individuals plan what types of meals they should be preparing in the coming days.

Exercise

People who have diabetes will benefit tremendously from physical exertion. Exercising burns fat! It is an important addition to a healthy lifestyle. Walking is a great form of exercise, and does not require any type of machinery to be executed. A simple walk around the block, or a long walk from the parking lot to the grocery store will do the trick! Making some changes in a person's diet and lifestyle will come a long way in the prevention of diabetes. These are just simple steps that can be done, but the benefits are immeasurable.

Discover the Link Between Obesity and Diabetes

Hyperglycemia, or escalated blood sugar levels is a characteristic that is linked with diabetes. This manifests itself through the symptoms of severe ongoing thirst, and constant need to urinate.

It is important to note that hyperglycemia is not always just linked with diabetes. It is a separate illness in itself.

Individuals who suffer from the symptoms of hyperglycemia should not automatically assume that they have diabetes. They should consult their physicians to get a proper diagnosis, and subsequent adequate treatment.

Type Two Diabetes

As discussed, this is the most common type of diabetes. The symptoms of this condition sometimes do not appear immediately. It could be years before an individual starts exhibiting symptoms related to this illness.

Also, This type of diabetes has been strongly attributed to genetics. Although, there are other factors that are connected to this disease such as: high blood pressure, a bad diet, sedentary lifestyle, and being overweight.

Obesity and type 2 Diabetes

Most individuals who are obese suffer from type 2 diabetes. It has been estimated that type 2 diabetes affect 80 percent of people who suffer from obesity.

But the positive thing about this is that it has been assessed that Type 2 Diabetes may be avoided and treated through a healthy lifestyle. Doctors ascribe a healthy and balanced diet in treating this type of diabetes.

Research has suggested that there's a strong link between obesity and diabetes. It is one of the main causes of type 2 diabetes.

In the United States one out of three of all Americans have been said to suffer from obesity. Type 2 diabetes does not only affect adults. During recent years there have been a rise in the number of children who are afflicted with this disease.

The problem with obesity is that in itself it is a serious health issue. People who suffer from obesity have a greater risk of developing high blood pressure, heart disease, liver disease, etc. This condition is also conducive to the onset of Type 2 diabetes.

Obesity is generally defined in individuals as having an unusually high proportion of body fat. Medical experts determine obesity by the amount of body mass a person has.

Causes of Obesity

Genetics- Medical experts have assessed that obesity has a strong link with genetics. Parents who are obese are more likely to have offspring who will be afflicted with obesity.

Although, it is not guaranteed that a person who has parents who suffer from obesity will have children who will also be afflicted with this condition.

Poor diet- Excessive consumption of foods that are high in calories can lead to obesity. Bad eating habits, and unregulated consumption of junk food such: candies, soft drinks, desserts, fast food meals can lead to excessive weight gain.

Alcohol- Excessive intake of alcohol can lead to obesity. It is extremely high in calories. Also, constant drinking of alcohol beverages promote appetite.

Smoking cigarettes- Smokers who have stopped smoking have a tendency to put on weight. Nicotine promotes the body's ability to burn calories. When nicotine stops going into their system, they tend to burn fewer calories; hence the weight gain.

Treatment

The positive news is recovering from obesity is possible. Shedding off some pounds can have tremendous benefits for those who are suffering from obesity. This will also greatly reduce the health risks that accompany this condition, including type 2 diabetes.

Changing to a healthier diet and exercising

Crash dieting to lose weight is never a good idea. In fact, this could lead to bigger problems. The lack of nutrient that goes into the body because of crash dieting can greatly harm the body!

Switching to fresh fruits and vegetables instead of foods rich in calories is the best way to start a healthy diet. Reducing the amount of calorie intake wlil also help in losing weight.

Also, never underestimate the benefits of exercising. Incorporating some physical activities to one's lifestyle will help tremendously in combating obesity.

It is never too late to become healthy. With the right amount of exercise and some dieting, people who suffer from obesity can improve their lifestyle today, and keeping diabetes at bay.

Diet and exercise for Diabetics

The best way to fight diabetes is through lifestyle changes particularly by combining diet and exercise. This is not new. Diabetes researchers and other experts have always suggested lifestyle changes as the major weapon in fighting diabetes. Studies have shown that people can greatly reduce their chances of acquiring diabetes if they exercise and follow a healthy diet. Overweight individuals can reduce their risk of getting diabetes by more than 50 percent if they could loose at least 10 pounds.

This brings good news to individuals with a moderate or high risk of getting diabetes. It means that the changes that need to be implemented are not big and drastic. One needs only to employ some little changes in his or her lifestyle in order to prevent diabetes. This is so empowering for individuals since it means that they have control over the dreaded disease.

Obese and overweight individuals actually have less insulin receptors than people with normal weights. This explains why most people with diabetes are either overweight or obese. Excess fat makes an individual's body insensitive to insulin. This means that overweight individuals need more insulin than people with normal weight. This is why reducing weight would greatly lower an individual's chance of getting diabetes.

Diet change: one of the best way to fight diabetes

The key is to combine exercise with proper diet. Proper diet here not only refers to reducing calorie intake. It also means eating the right kind of food. One should avoid foods that are rich in fat particularly animal fat. They should also lessen their intake of red meat, dairy products and eggs. Processed and refined carbohydrates are big no-nos. These include refined sugar, white rice and white flour. Instead, one should consume whole grains like millet rice and unrefined rice (brown or red) and whole wheat.

There are foods that have an insulin-like effect in the body when consumed. Some examples of these are: cucumbers, garlic, soy, wheat germ, avocados, green beans, buckwheat, flaxseed oil, green vegetables (raw) and Brussels sprout. People who believe that they are at risk of getting diabetes must increase their consumption of these foods.

Intake of fiber can also greatly reduce the risk of diabetes. High fiber foods are usually low in sugar. Individuals with diabetes or at risk of getting diabetes cannot process sugar properly. Individuals who are at risk of getting diabetes are advised to increase their fiber intake by taking fiber supplements such as guar gum, psyllium, oat bran or glucomannan. They should also consume more vegetables, fruits, whole wheat products and whole grain products. Intake of white sugar and foods high with it must be cut. You must replace these foods with ones that have high fiber content.

People should also stay away from alcoholic drinks if they really want to avoid having diabetes. Alcohol decreases glucose tolerance especially in the elderly and those already at high risk of getting diabetes. Moreover, diabetics who consume even moderate quantities of alcoholic drinks have a great risk of damaging their eyes and nerves. Apart from alcoholic drinks, smoking must also be avoided to be safe from getting diabetes. Cigarettes increases the risk for heart disease, kidney problems and other health concerns connected to diabetes. Heavy smokers are more likely to become diabetics than non-smokers. So if you are currently it is of your best interest to quit the habit. If you don't smoke then just don't pick up the habit.

Exercise protects you from diabetes

Both type 1 and 2 diabetes can be avoided and improved with a regular moderate exercise regimen. In fact, individuals with type 1 diabetes who exercise regularly require less insulin while healthy individuals who exercise regularly are less likely to develop type 2 diabetes. This is because working out reduces the amount of body fat and thus improves the sensitivity of the body to insulin.

The exercises need not be strenuous. Simple aerobic activities like walking, running, swimming and cycling can greatly improve blood sugar levels. Exercise improves the utilization of glucose by the muscles involved. This effect can last up to more than two days. Blood fat profile and blood pressure which also affects diabetes also improves with regular exercise.

Individuals, especially those who are already diabetic, must monitor their blood sugar level when exercising. This is because exercise can either increase or decrease blood sugar. It is always advisable to ask your physician before going into an exercise program.

Remember, if you think you have Diabetes or have been recently diagnosed, consult with your physician to conduct the necessary tests. Consult with a qualified nutritionist who specializes in diabetes management for a more personalized nutrition and wellness protocol..

www.ingramcontent.com/pod-product-compliance
Lightning Source LLC
Chambersburg PA
CBHW070228210526
45169CB00023B/1459